The Smart & Easy Guide To Yoga: The Ultimate Yoga Book For Workouts, Diet, Poses, Sequencing, Practice, Philosophy & Life

Swami Bhajan

I0415627

Legal Stuff

Table of Contents

The Enjoyment of Yoga

The unification of the mind, body and spirit is a common purpose among yoga practitioners. Achieving this unification is easy as long as one practices yoga techniques and exercises.

In yoga, the mind and body being unified is already considered a fundamental belief. One's body can easily find harmony and even heal itself when put into a proper environment. Due to this belief, yoga is now a popular therapy that even doctors recommend. It provides reliable results while curing nervous system illnesses.

Yoga has been in existence ever since ancient times. Since it has been practiced for a long period of time, a lot of people have benefitted from its reliable results. There are even investigations done just to establish the excellent health results of the said practice. The results of such an investigation can be divided into the physiological, psychological and biochemical categories.

In terms of the physiological aspects, the practice of yoga cures dysfunction in the respiratory system, pulse rate, and blood pressure. It easily contributes to the stabilization of the equilibrium of the nervous system and normalization of gastrointestinal and endocrine functions. Aside from that, yoga helps increase joint range of motion, disease immunity, cardiovascular efficiency, endurance level and energy level. It also improves reaction time, depth perception, dexterity skills, eye-to-hand coordination and other similar skills.

In terms of the psychological aspects, yoga contributes to an increase of self-acceptance, somatic awareness, kinesthetic awareness, self-actualization and well-being. It is also known to increase social skills as well as improve one's learning efficiency, attention, concentration, memory and other similar skills.

For the biochemical aspects, enumerating the benefits of yoga is easy as well. Expect a significant decrease in the level of cholesterol, sodium, white blood cells and glucose in the body. It will also promote an increase in the levels of hemoglobin, serum protein and vitamin C.

The benefits of yoga do not end there. Yoga is also known to be effective in increasing the joint flexibility level as well as levels of lubrication for ligaments, joints and tendons. Practicing yoga can help massage the glands and internal organs of the body too. Even those organs that one rarely uses will be stimulated properly with yoga. If the organs of the body are properly stimulated and massaged, it should help keep any kind of disease away.

Another benefit of yoga is that it can be used to detoxify the body. Yoga requires the person to stretch the muscles and massage the joints. The complexity of this exercise will really ensure that the body receives the maximum blood supply it needs. This means that the toxins in the body are effectively eliminated and natural body processes like aging are delayed.

The aforementioned benefits are advantages that one can enjoy only when one practices yoga. Of course, these benefits are reaped together with the main benefit of yoga which is the unification of the mind, body and spirit. It should also be obvious that yoga strengthens the meditation and emotional systems that one has.

How to Get Started with Yoga

It is a known fact that yoga produces great benefits without incurring any costs. This is a kind of relaxation technique that does not even require any specific training equipment. There is no need to order anything just to get good results since the person can practice yoga anytime and anywhere.

Unlike normal exercises, yoga is not just a practice. It is more like a lifestyle for some and a state of mind for others. As long as the person has the will to practice yoga along with the appropriate belief and attitude toward the practice, good results will be obtained. The person should also have a balanced diet based on natural foods to prepare for the first session of yoga practice. The food one eats affects both the mind and soul so pay attention to it.

Remember that there is no special environment for practicing yoga. However, the person should be prudent enough to choose a place where there are no distractions such as street noise or radio. It should also be a clean, quiet place that has proper ventilation. Since yoga involves various sitting and lying positions, obtaining a blanket, a mat or a towel should be beneficial.

What one wears while practicing yoga will also matter. The person has to feel comfortable so select something that is both comfortable and loose. The best options are sweatpants, training suits, t-shirts, shorts or loose pajamas. If the person is doing a yoga session alone in a private space, then it is fine to practice yoga naked if one prefers to do so.

Practicing yoga on an empty stomach is actually recommended. This is why it is the most ideal to practice yoga at least an hour or two after eating a main meal. Also, cleaning the throat and nostrils is important since breathing is a vital element for a yoga exercise.

There may be times when the person cannot decide what time of the day they should practice yoga. Regardless of whether the person chooses morning or evening, remember that practicing yoga gives the same benefits to the body and mind. Practicing yoga in the morning will result in a good mood the entire day. On the other hand, practicing yoga in the evening promotes a good night's sleep.

The yoga exercise should not be exhausting. This means that you can easily take a break when you are already feeling tired. It is common for a yoga session to allow the participants to have short breaks, especially in between the difficult exercises. As long as the person has gone through at least 15 minutes of proper yoga exercise, the body and mind will already receive significant results.

In practicing yoga, you will have to remember a vital key point. This is that your attitude towards the said practice is very important. Aside from that, you should have the desire to discover new sensations and fresh experiences with yoga.

What Diet to Follow for Yoga

In yoga, having a positive attitude is vital. In addition, it is also important to have a balanced diet. It is recommended to practice yoga one to two hours after eating a main meal, when the stomach is already empty. For the yoga specialists, they will certainly agree that the food we eat will affect our appearance. It will also affect our health. These are the reasons why it is necessary to pay attention to what we consume to prevent diseases.

The question is, what kind of healthy food should people consume? This is a usual inquiry that people make when they are told to have a balanced meal. Nowadays, there are studies that show it is ideal for people to have a diversified diet. While that might be the case, there is an emphasis on having fruits and vegetables as a staple part of the diet because of their vitamins and fibers. In addition, all natural foods are recommended to preserve your health.

Some people might prefer to eat less than normal because they believe that eating food will cause them harm. Instead of this train of thought, you should replace this with the fact that the body needs the food to supply the nutrients the body requires to function properly. Do not overeat, though, even if the foods are all natural. Overdoing it will really cause problems. The limit to one's appetite should be when one is not hungry anymore. Even better, it is recommended to stop eating before you reach your full saturation state. That way you will not feel fatigued even after eating a substantial amount of food and increasing your energy level.

It is necessary for you to establish how often you should eat. Also, better determine if it is okay to have three meals daily. Consider the pros and cons of skipping any meals too, regardless of whether the meal is breakfast, lunch or dinner. Otherwise, you might not have sufficient flexibility. If you are confused and cannot establish a reasonable answer, better remember that it is more suitable for the person to eat when hungry than to be able to move. However, pay attention to what and how much one should eat.

Food is more than a source of energy. It can also help purify the body and spirit. This is why it is appropriate to eat a balanced diet when doing yoga exercises. A yoga trainer will even recommend this, with emphasis on natural food in the diet. This should prevent the body from contracting diseases and toxins. It will also help in performing yoga and unifying the spirit and mind.

If the person has a goal of performing yoga exercises, it is necessary to meditate on what one is doing to the body. Remember that the body is a reflection of one's diet. Aside from that, establish the response level that one should have for the needs of the spirit and mind.

What Equipment to Use for Yoga

Preparing for the practice of yoga is easy. You should follow a proper diet. Also, you should prepare mentally for practicing yoga. There are a few easy-to-obtain exercise tools that you need to get. Obtaining these exercise tools is optional but recommended because they increase comfort and efficiency. Here are the things to keep in mind when deciding on an exercise tool.

1. Yoga clothing. In performing yoga techniques and exercises, there is no strict rule to follow for clothing. However, there is an appropriate outfit that you should opt for. You should wear comfortable, loose and well-ventilated materials because they are convenient for this practice. Sweatsuits or loose pajamas are often preferred. If you follow a regular routine that includes the head coming below the knees, a T-shirt that s tightly to the body is the best choice.

2. Shoes. A general rule in performing yoga is that you should do it without any footwear. People's shoes are usually left at a shoe rack by the entrance. If you are uncomfortable coming into direct contact with the cold floor, put on light cotton socks.

3. Blankets. Piles of blankets will become useful during a yoga session. A yoga studio will have a pile of blankets prepared for every yoga session so one should grab one. The blankets can help as props when performing a routine involving an uncomfortable position. It can be used to cover yourself when you are relaxing at the end of a routine too.

4. Mats. A yoga room will usually have a large number of mats spread out on the floor. The mats are there to distinguish the space dedicated to each individual. This is the space allocated to every individual where they can practice yoga without bothering anyone. It is also the space that only you can inhabit. With the mats, you should be able to attain a certain level of comfort for the practice. They also promote stability, especially when you become sweaty to the point that it is possible to slip because of your sweat. The mats should help you stay focused in such situations. Getting a mat is especially recommended for beginners since this also prevents the discomfort caused by the hard floor. Some yoga studios may rent yoga mats for a cheap price. However, it is still better to purchase your own yoga mat.

There are still other elements to use for the yoga routine. For example, you will also need some straps ad blocks to carry out some yoga positions. The blocks and straps should help increase comfort and efficiency.

How to Correctly Do the Breathing Techniques for Yoga Exercises

A yoga routine can be carried out whenever you want or wherever you are. However, there are some details, like what you ate before you came to the yoga studio and such, which will affect your breathing techniques and even your attitude towards yoga.

Things like breathing are a vital element that will certainly make a difference in every yoga session that you participate in. First of all, you should know how to breathe properly during yoga so that you can supply your body with the right amount of oxygen necessary to survive. Another importance of the breathing process is that it is very efficient in getting rid of body toxins.

Just like flowers require water to develop and grow, what humans essentially need to survive is oxygen. Not only is it important for the nervous system, it is also necessary for a series of glands and internal organs. The most important organ that will require a consistent supply of oxygen is the brain. If it does not receive its required supply of oxygen, it might cause damage not only to your brain but to your other organs too.

After determining the importance of having enough oxygen supply to the body, it is only natural to consider what the best breathing techniques are. While breathing in itself is a natural process of the body, you should still be able to modify or restrict it in some ways. There are actions you can perform. However, these actions may cause negative effects when done incorrectly. Even in daily living, you might have to assume some positions or actions which diminish your lung capacity which, in turn, also makes the interval for breathing a lot shorter.

The manner by which you breathe will have a close connection to your mental state. That is why it is only appropriate to learn more about the proper breathing techniques to assume when one is practicing yoga so that you can achieve a good harmony between your body and spirit. With proper execution of these breathing techniques, you can easily reach a desired peaceful stage. The breathing techniques also promote synchronization between the inner and outer self.

The breathing techniques used in yoga are not fast and shallow. It is, in fact, the opposite of that. Yoga uses deep breathing, since it promotes a variety of benefits. Here are some of the important benefits of deep breathing.

1. Improvement of your oxygen irrigation system for the body and brain.

2. Rejuvenation of your skin and gradual elimination of facial wrinkles, which promotes smoother skin.

3. Improvement of lung capacity and heart health, making both stronger and healthier.

4. Relaxation of both the mind and body.

Breathing Techniques for Yoga: What is Pranayama?

If you cannot use the proper breathing techniques while doing yoga, your exercises are no more than acrobatics. The breathing techniques allow you to optimize the full benefits of yoga as well as bring a new way for you to perceive life. Inhaling oxygen helps your body absorb the nutrients you eat. Exhaling will eliminate unwanted carbon dioxide which is toxic for the body.

Prana is the yoga term referring to life force. This is the combination of attributes from the elemental spheres of both your physiological and spiritual aspects. What fuels this life force is air. That is the reason why one should master both the input and output of air to maximize the positive effects of yoga exercises. Bear in mind that the breathing techniques will contribute to your mental status as well. Fast and irregular breathing will stress the mind and make it anxious. On the other hand, deep breathing will bring stillness and increase concentration.

Yoga stresses maximizing the various benefits of *prana*. This is where the art of mastering breathing comes in. This art is called *pranayama*, which helps you achieve above-average results for the mind and body. *Pranayama* is a part of the preparation exercises for different yoga poses. It helps achieve a superior state of mind, allowing your body to practice yoga as much as you can.

Breathing Techniques for Yoga: What is Anuloma Viloma?

Anuloma Viloma is commonly known as the technique of Alternate Nostril Breathing. Most practitioners of yoga inhale through only one nostril, then retain the breath for some time, and then use the other nostril to exhale. The left nostril is a path of the *Nadi* known as *Ida*. The right nostril is a path of the *Nadi* known as *Pingala*. For a healthy person, breathing through *Ida* is possible for approximately two hours, followed by *Pingala*.

It is just unfortunate that most people's breathing rhythm is actually disturbed. This is precarious to your health. This is where Anuloma Viloma comes in. It restores, equalizes and slowly balances *prana* flow in your body.

There are steps to follow for Anuloma Viloma. Here are the six steps.

1. Tuck both your index and middle finger into the nostril to close it. The thumb should be positioned to the right while the ring finger and little finger are positioned on the left. First inhale through the left nostril. Keep the right nostril closed with the thumb. Count one to four while keeping this position.

2. Hold that breath you inhaled up to a count of 16.

3. Exhale that breath through the right nostril to a count of eight. Close the left nostril.

4. This time, inhale through the right nostril. Keep the left nostril closed. Count one to four.

5. Hold your breath and then count to 16.

6. Exhale through the left nostril for a count of eight. Close the right nostril.

Breathing Techniques for Yoga: What is Ujjayi?

Ujjayi is known to be a loud breathing technique. This is usually performed by breathing through both of your nostrils. While breathing, the glottis should be kept closed to a certain degree. This breathing technique should increase your control over your lung activity. It helps clear the throat as well. *Ujjayi* involves air passing through a partially closed glottis, which makes a constant, fluent sound. A yoga practitioner attempts to eliminate any nasal sound and keep a constant air and sound flow to promote harmony.

To practice *Ujjayi*, a chin lock is necessary to ensure the closure of your nostrils. Hold your breath for as long as possible. At the end, gently exhale. In this breathing technique, the left nostril will be used when exhaling. If the person has kept the left nostril closed, just release it and the air will naturally flow out. Release the pressure put on both the nostrils so that you can unlock your chin and open your glottis to a greater extent.

Inhaling should be half of the time reserved for exhaling. Each person might have different moments for both inhalation and exhalation so better find them out personally while practicing this breathing technique. Holding your breath for a long time might be difficult. However, you will certainly get used to this and even extend your time when you use *Ujjayi* repeatedly.

The Pose Sequence for Every Yoga Session

In order to maximize the results of yoga, it is recommended to use a good practice rhythm. This means that you need to perform *asanas* in the correct order to find out your rhythm. It will also allow you to flow from one stage of yoga to another without any interruptions. The initial pose for yoga is the corpse pose. This used repeatedly between other *asanas* as well as your final relaxation method. The easy pose is a standard pose in yoga. It is perfect to recharge energy. It is an excellent position to be in for meditation too. It allows the brain to gain strength. When using the easy position, mind your back position to prevent it from arching.

Continue with your warm up exercises. Try to relax the neck muscles, as this is the upper point of the body's central line represented by the spinal cord. Shoulder lifts come next.

Try a few of the eye exercises in yoga as well, to prevent tiredness and improve eyesight strength. The sun salutation pose, which stretches all body muscles, should be assumed as well in preparation for those difficult *asanas*. If you want to tone your leg muscles to improve flexibility and endurance, leg raises are appropriate. On the other hand, those who want to rest specific body organs like the heart should consider the head stand pose. A good variation to this is the shoulder stand. It is beneficial to lower back and spinal muscles.

Use the bridge and plough poses to increase back flexibility. They might look difficult to perform but they are both accessible using gentle movements. You might not achieve a perfect stance even after a few attempts. Do not get discouraged by this. After all, it will take time to develop the flexibility and strength for the proper execution of these poses. The forward bend pose should help stimulate your nervous system. The fish pose, although rather acrobatic, helps tone lungs and chest muscles. Women suffering from various menstrual problems can try the cobra position. It stimulates both the lower abdomen and pelvic area, which improves circulation and massages internal organs.

The locust pose can strengthen the lower back. It also has positive effects on the abdominal muscles. Not only that, it prevents constipation. Another pose is the bow. It helps the back area remain strong and flexible. Most abdominal fat can be reduced with the bow pose, as long as you follow a proper diet. The half spine twist pose can further the exercise routine for the spine too.

The crow pose helps improve arm and joint strength. It will positively affect your breathing since your chest area is forced to expand, providing better breathing capabilities. The hands-to-feet pose and triangle pose test the strength and flexibility of your body as well. Lastly, the final corpse pose helps the body rest and recharge energy lost during yoga practice.

What are the Prone Yoga Poses?

Before practicing yoga, it is necessary to start warming up with some easy positions. A single leg raise should start the yoga session and will prepare you for the next poses. With leg raises, you can improve your abdominal and back muscles tone. To effectively do leg raises, make sure to hold your back to the floor. The spine should not bend. The shoulders should help with the lifting motion as well. The palms should remain on the floor. After these preparations, raise the legs slowly. During the motion, keep the neck relaxed and the lungs breathing freely.

If the person wants to improve leg muscles and their flexibility, the leg pull is a good choice. This will give a complete stretch to the leg muscles. When done properly, it helps you over time to move into performing advanced *asanas*. While on the floor, catch your foot so that your leg is straight above your head. Those having problems with this can use a belt for assistance. Remember to keep the leg straight. Point the heel upward, toward the ceiling. Pull the leg close to the body but the back should be straight and the shoulders should be close to the floor. Slide the other leg on the floor. Make sure to straighten it. Roll the thigh until the kneecap is faced toward the ceiling. Press your feet away from you, all the while keeping the shoulders flat, and spread them. The raised leg should then be pulled toward you.

Remember that your movement and breathing control is vital in yoga. To get ready, try to use *Bidalasana*. This is also known as the cat pose. With this technique, both balance and coordination can be improved. Your body center's alignment will be corrected, making it relative to the central area's position. The hip area should be the central balance pose for all *asanas* since it dictates the direction and movement of the spine. For the cat tilt pose, the hip should be bent forward to make the spine arch backward. If the person does not want the cat tilt pose, use the dog tilt. Some poses might require neutral choices but some will require a combination.

Yoga Exercises: What is the Cat Pose?

Yoga poses exist to prepare the body muscles for better flexibility and strength. Muscle stretches help not only with your performance of yoga poses but with blood circulation as well. They stimulate nerve endings which keep the body alive and energetic. Prone poses should teach you how to get a good yoga posture, straightening the back. There are poses that might be demanding at the beginning. However, you will surely get better at them over time.

Yoga Exercises: What is the Corpse Pose?

The corpse pose is a classic relaxation pose in yoga. It is also a difficult yoga pose to execute. This pose should be practiced before *asanas*, between *asanas*, or during final relaxation.

Before executing this pose, the body should be laid out symmetrically. This is so that you can have enough space for stretching the hands and legs. After successfully completing this pose, you will feel that your muscles are relaxed.

To execute this pose, start by rotating the legs. Let them fall to the sides slowly. Repeat the said movement with the hands. The next move is for the spine. First, rotate the head from side to side. Stretch the body as much as possible, as if someone is trying to pull the head and feet apart. The shoulders should be down but away from the feet.

This should relax the body. Remember to pay attention to the breathing technique one uses for yoga. Breathe deeply so that the abdomen rises while you inhale. When doing this pose, the entire body goes through a variety of beneficial actions. It should help remove stress and reduce energy loss.

Among the many poses, the corpse pose is still the most popular one in relaxation poses.

Yoga Exercises: What is the Easy Pose?

This is another relaxation pose which is normally used after the corpse pose.

The easy pose is commonly known as *Sukhasana*. It is a great pose for meditation. You just need to sit down, bend the knees, and then clasp the arms around the knees. You need to press them until you reach your chest. The spine should be straight by then. When done, release the arms and place the legs in a crossing position. It is fine to let the knees fall down on the floor. Just make sure to put the hands on top of your knees, with the palms facing upward.

The head should be kept up and the spine's position should be straight. It is important to pay attention to breathing. Make sure to fill the lungs with air and hold it. Remember to breathe through the nose. When doing the easy pose, relax the face, especially the belly and jaws.

The good thing about the easy pose is that it is a good frequent practice. It is good for people coming from any age group as well. However, the easy pose should be avoided when one receives a knee injury or inflammation. It will be uncomfortable. It is okay to put a folded blanket under the hip bones or knees to increase the comfort level.

This is a pose that is good for meditation. It is recommended because it is easy to perform. It also promotes relaxation and inner calm.

Yoga Exercises: What is the Cobra Pose?

The cobra pose is a yoga pose which will require the head and trunk to arch up gracefully. Stretch the spine and abdominal organs together, along with the nearby musculature to get a massage. With this pose, one can obtain relief against pain, constipation and even menstrual irregularities.

To execute the said exercise, keep the shoulders down. The face should be relaxed while the elbows are comfortably tucked to the body. Lie down, making sure that the legs are together. Place the palms under the shoulders and rest the forehead on the floor.

When you are inhaling, move the head slowly upwards. Brush the nose first against the mat followed by the chin. Lift the hands, all the while making sure to use the back muscles. This should raise the chest high. Hold your breath for several seconds and then exhale to slowly return to your initial position.

When the person is gradually returning to your initial position, use the hands to push your trunk upward. The body should be pushed upward, to attempt to bend from the center of the spine. Hold this position for at most three breaths. Exhale while slowly coming down.

Raise the trunk again, not forgetting to inhale deeply. Bend the back this time until it bends from the neck to the spine's base. Hold this position as long as you are comfortable. Breathe normally, and then slowly return to your initial position. Relax.

Yoga Exercises: What Is The Bow Pose?

One of the yoga exercises to follow is the bow pose. This involves raising the upper and lower half of the body at the same time. To form the curve necessary for the bow pose, use the hands and arms to pull the trunks and legs up. This movement will tone the back muscles and increase the spine's elasticity. It also increases vitality and improves posture. The bow pose aims to balance the weight of the body on the abdomen. This is the best way to reduce abdominal fat and massage internal organs.

To form the bow pose, you need to lie on your front comfortably while keeping the head down. While inhaling, bring the knees up and then reach back using your hands to hold the ankles. Remain in this position and then exhale. Inhale deeply while simultaneously raising the head and chest and pulling the ankles up. Do not look down when arching backwards. Maintain this position and then take three slow, deep breaths. Exhale and release the ankles.

The person may perform the rocking bow pose after executing this bow position. When in the bow position, gradually rock backward and forward. Do not forget to exhale when rocking forward and inhale when rocking backward. The head should be stationary when doing the rocking bow pose. Do not look down. Repeat this ten times before completely relaxing the body.

Yoga Exercise: What is the Shoulder Stand?

The shoulder stand is a good yoga *asana* that is popular with most practitioners. This pose requires deep breathing if you do not want this to become just an acrobatic position. Many gyms and sports training facilities adopt the shoulder stand pose because of its efficiency. It can be done by both male and female practitioners.

To begin, lie on your back. The legs should be kept straight and close to one another while the arms are parallel to the torso. Raise the legs toward the ceiling while pointing the toes upward. The weight of the body should be resting on the neck muscles and shoulder's deltoid muscles. Do not forget to move the legs and back into a vertical position by simply using the hands to give balance to the lower back. Remember to take deep breaths when executing this pose.

Hold the shoulder stand pose with the legs. Keep the spine straight. After that, take slow, deep breaths while focusing on your thyroid gland. The thyroid gland is found in the neck area. This pose will increase the tone -n this area. Remember to keep this pose for several minutes to get good effects.

To wrap up this position, curve the knees and back at the same time, then lower them to the floor. Remove your hands from their position and then place them flat on the ground. Straighten the knees and then lower the legs gently when your back is already completely flat on the floor.

Yoga Exercise: What is the Fish Pose?

The fish pose is actually considered the natural successor of the shoulder stand pose. It is recommended for people to practice this as a counter pose to the shoulder stand. This pose involves a proper compression of the neck and spine. This is quite the opposite of the stretching obtained using the shoulder stand or any other poses such as bridge or plough poses.

Know that there are numerous benefits to the fish pose. The first benefit you can enjoy is the expansion of the chest cavity. This enables your lungs to breathe more air. You will also become more used to any deep breathing techniques for yoga this way. The fish pose will also help make the nerves and neck muscles stronger. They will be more responsive, especially when the spine increases flexibility.

To begin this pose, you will have to lie down on your back. Your legs should be kept close to one another and straight out. The spine should also be kept straight and parallel to the ground. It is important to pay attention to the position of your arms. The arms should be straight and then positioned under your thighs. Your palms should rest together while held to the ground. The elbows should be as close to one another as possible.

Pressing the elbows down onto the floor, while arching the back, is how you begin this pose. Do not forget to take deep breaths. The weight of the entire body should be kept on the elbows. After that, your head should be moved backwards gently until it reaches the ground. Upon reaching the peak, breathe out while holding the pose. Keep the legs relaxed. Allow the chest to gently expand, especially when taking in long breaths. If you are planning to come out of this pose, lift your head slowly. After that, release the pressure you have been putting on your elbows.

Yoga Exercise: What is the Leg Raise?

One of the easy yoga poses you can take advantage of these days is the leg raise. This is an exercise which actually has a goal of preparing your body to various yoga *asanas*. With the leg raises, you can easily straighten and tone both your lower back muscles and abdominal muscles.. It is also the best way to tone the leg muscles. Those people who do not have strong muscles might find this exercise a little bit difficult to execute in the beginning. It will get easier as one carries out the leg raise pose repeatedly.

If you are not in your best condition you might need to use your shoulders or arch your lower back just to help you lift your legs. You should maximize the effects of this pose, and the best recommendation for this is to have the entire length of the body resting on the floor. Both your back and shoulders should be relaxed. To begin the leg raises, position the legs together. Your palms should also be on the sides of your body.

The leg raises can be done by either just raising one leg while the other remains on the ground or raising both legs simultaneously. If you plan to work with only one leg, then push down with your hands to easily facilitate leg lifting. The best results can be achieved if the knees are maintained straight. The back should be lowered down onto the floor to straighten your spine.

When executing this pose, you will have to remember the breathing techniques you have learned. It is a widely known fact that deep breathing will easily contribute to immediate and satisfying results.

Yoga Exercise: What is the Bridge Pose?

The bridge pose will be accomplished when you come down from a shoulder stand pose. For this, the feet will be going in opposite directions. Your spine will be experiencing a reverse bend and all pressure will be relieved from the neck. If the person holds this bridge pose, it will benefit the abdominal and back muscles a lot. The pose will surely help you develop a more flexible spine as well as stronger wrists. Be cautious and keep the thumbs pointed in a similar direction as your shoulder stand pose. If you are not cautious, you might end up hurting your fingers.

The first thing for executing this bridge pose is to lie on your back as an initial position. Hold the feet together and keep your knees bent too. In the same manner as with the shoulder stand, lift the hips as far out as possible. You should place your hands on your lower back. The shoulder stand will help prepare for the bridge, reversing all pose movements until one completes the shoulder stand pose. After executing the bridge pose over and over again, go back to the shoulder stand position. Bend the right leg while you are lowering it to the ground.

Your left leg should be brought down then, together with the right. You should maintain this bridge pose by inhaling deeply several times. Then, take one deep breath and then go into the shoulder stand pose. Release the pose to come out of it. After doing this over and over, you will start noticing how it is possible to lower both of your legs at the same time. It might be a difficult pose if you do not have enough spinal flexibility. However, this will be easily achieved if one is willing to execute the said pose repeatedly.

Yoga Exercise: What is the Plow Pose?

If you will execute the plow pose, you will need to use flexibility and your muscle tone and flexibility. Your flexibility and muscle tone can be developed through other yoga *asanas*, like the shoulder stand. If a person practices a lot, then it will be easy to execute the plow pose with grace.

The person will start from the shoulder stand when executing the plow pose. Then lower the feet onto the ground slowly, just above your head. Remember to keep your legs extended all the time. The position of your spinal column will have to be perpendicular to the ground. Hold your toes to the floor and continue raising your lower back and pelvis, aiming for the ceiling.

Pay attention to the position of your head and neck. Keep the neck as relaxed as possible and your muscles soft. Your chin should be pressed away from your chest, to make the relaxation easier. After that, press the arms down to the ground. This will serve as your support since you will need to hold this pose. Remember that your hands will have to be pressed to your lower back area to push it towards the ceiling.

There are many variations to the said pose. You can do it by simply releasing the lower back and then moving the hands opposite to your legs and onto the floor. Press both your lower arm and palms on the ground to attempt to push the thighs higher up, towards the ceiling.

Get out of the said pose. You can do this by bringing your arms down to your lower back region. Roll out of the said pose. Do not forget to exhale while executing this pose.

Yoga Exercise: What is the Locust Pose?

The locust pose is one excellent pose in yoga that should help improve the lower back muscles' strength. Aside from that, it will be useful for toning both the leg and arms muscles. The locust should allow you to prepare your body for the difficult bending poses that you will need to execute later on. Some people might dismiss the locust pose as simple-looking. If the truth be told, it has a certain degree of difficulty which will certainly challenge and reward a practitioner.

The said pose has numerous benefits. One benefit is the improvement of your back position and posture, both when you are standing and walking. It is recommended to attempt to execute this pose when the body is in its best condition. Be sure to be extremely careful when executing this pose if you have suffered from neck or back injuries.

To begin this locust pose, lie on your front while keeping your hands close to your body. Your palms should be facing up while resting on the ground. By moving your big toes so that they face one another, you will be rotating your thighs inward. Remember your breathing techniques as well. When exhaling, you should move both your legs and arms away from the ground. Your upper body, along with your head, should move in an upward direction while keeping your belly's balance even.

You should stretch your arms. Remember to keep them in a parallel position to the floor. After that, you will have to press your arms upward. Do not forget to keep the base of your head lifted since it will be useful in a slightly raised position. Hold the said pose. It might be difficult after one holds it for a while. Just make sure to hold this pose for a minute. Exhale while coming out of the pose. Of course it is also important to rest and take deep breaths before executing the said pose again.

Yoga Exercise: What Are the Best Yoga Standing Poses?

In yoga, lying down or sitting can be effective positions. However, the most efficient poses are usually the standing ones. They offer excellent muscle stretching, and usually have a significant effect on the nervous system. Using standing poses allows you to have improved *asanas*. It also offers increased chances for mastering a proper equilibrium between your physical and mental aspects. The standing poses should improve the *asanas*. To those who want to benefit from this, here are some of the things to know.

First is the mountain pose, also known as *Tadasana*. This pose got its name from its defining attributes which basically share mountain symbols. One can benefit a lot from this pose, specifically because it gives you an invulnerable feeling and relaxed strength just like a mountain. You will be surrounded by a feeling of stillness and balance. With the clarity and vision provided by the mountain pose, you can easily dig deeper into your inner feelings. You can easily establish a connection with your inner pose.

To go through with the mountain pose, you need to keep your heels slightly apart, the toes parallel to one another. Execute a back and forth rocking motion, stressing the weight on the toes, and then gradually come to a complete stop. Next, lift your ankles while tightening your leg muscles, to strengthen your pose. Your tailbones should then be pushed towards the floor, all the while lifting the pelvic area toward your navel. Be sure to have your arms hanging near the body, all the while pressing the shoulder blades backwards.

It should be obvious that the mountain pose will benefit you since it becomes the basis for the other poses. This pose just implies that yoga is for learning the proper meaning of stillness and balance. This is certainly an effective way to establish connection with your inner self all the while learning the various ways of yoga.

The person should also take advantage of another standing pose. This is the triangle pose, better known as *trikonasana*. This is an easy pose which will produce a stretching effect on your spine. The pose has a lateral motion that properly complements any stretching motion for the other forward poses. This will usually involve keeping the knees straight, which becomes vital to the execution of the pose. This allows you to have a fluent movement and to stretch all of your targeted organs and muscles. This kind of yoga standing pose requires you to bend left and right as well, gradually and fluently. If done properly, it should easily prepare you for the next posture levels, especially with the more advanced and difficult poses. With the *trikonasana*, you can stimulate your spinal nerves and benefit from improved total body flexibility.

To be able to enjoy the triangle pose, make sure to have the body positioned correctly. Spread your feet apart while pointing to your toes. It will be more appropriate to try out an alternate pointing motion, starting from the left foot to the right. Keep a constant rhythm for this along with a perfect balance as well. Stretch your arms, which are parallel to the floor. After that, take a deep breath and draw energy from it to strengthen your body movements. Once you release your breath, execute a slight bend. You can choose to do it to the left or you might prefer the right. While bending, slide down your hand to your foot. With this motion, your flexibility within your lower back muscle area will be tested. This action will certainly become a good warmup session and is absolutely necessary for performing the triangle pose. If done successfully, it will give a feeling of lightness to the body. There is also the nice sensation of mild heat within your stretched muscles.

Yoga Exercise: What is the Sun Salutation

The sun salutation is a pose that is highly recommended for yoga practitioners coming from any age bracket. It is especially recommended for those who do not have sufficient time to dedicate to practicing a yoga routine. The said pose should allow you to enjoy stimulation for all muscle groups and even the respiratory system.

Remember that the sun salutation has twelve yoga positions put into a sequence and linked together using a flowing motion. It is also being accompanied by five deep and special breaths. The twelve yoga positions are said to contribute in stretching different muscle groups and body parts. Aside from that, these positions are said to help with the expansion and contraction of the chest, which basically helps in regulating your breathing.

Those who are knowledgeable in yoga will certainly recommend this as an exercise on a daily basis. It will contribute in an efficient manner to your spine and joint flexibility, after all.

1. The first position to hold when executing the sun salutation requires you to stand up, feet together. Put your palms together in front of the chest in a praying position. Make sure to evenly distribute your weight. After this, exhale.

2. Inhale. While doing so, you should then push your arms up. Do not forget to keep your legs straight. Also remember to relax your neck.

3. Exhale. While doing so, you should then fold the body forward. After that, press the palms down, placing your fingertips in the same line as your toes.

4. Inhale again. This time, you should bring your leg back in place to the floor while inhaling. You should then arch the back and lift your chin.

5. Bring your other leg back in. This time you can support your weight using your hands and toes. You should then keep your chin down so that you can retain your breathing while executing this action.

6. Exhale again. While exhaling, you should lower your knees first, followed by the forehead. Remember to keep the hips up. Make sure to keep the toes curled under as well.

7. Inhale. While doing so, you should lower your hips. After that, point the toes and then bend back as much as you can. The shoulders must be kept down, while keeping your legs together.

8. Exhale. Your toes should be curled under too. Raise your hips after that. The form that you should assume during this action is a V position. Push both your head and heels down. Remember to keep your shoulders back.

9. Inhale. You should then step forward, placing one leg between your hands. You should keep your chin up while your other knee is resting on the ground.

10. Your other leg should be brought forward. Slowly bend down from your waist while keeping your palms pressed on the floor. Exhale.

11. This time, you will take a deep breath again. Stretch the arms forward, up, and then back over to your head. You should then try to bend back slowly and gently.

12. When done, return to your original upright standing position. Exhale. While doing so, bring the arms to your sides.

Yoga Exercise: What is the Crow Pose?

With the crow pose for yoga, you will be using your elbows to support your entire body weight, all the while keeping your head and hands oriented forward. It is not difficult to accomplish this pose as long as you bend forward enough so that it prevents your strength from wandering. You should execute the crow pose regularly to benefit from it through strengthened shoulders, arms and wrists. Your concentration level will also be improved as well as your breathing capacity expanded.

If you want to execute this pose, start by squatting down. Bring the arms in between the knees. The palms should then be positioned down on the ground, in front of the body. The shoulders should be apart while your fingers are pointing slightly inwards. After you get into the said position, slowly bend the elbows out to your sides. This means that you will be converting the back of the arms into a comfortable shelf for the knees. You should look forward. It is also required to breathe normally when executing this pose.

Once you are in this position, identify a single reference point in front of you. This might be a part of the ground or the wall. You will be focusing on this reference point while doing the pose. Be careful with your breathing technique since it will be vital in this phase. Inhale so that you can easily retain your breath. While retaining a deep breath, you should lean forward to your reference point. When doing this, you will have to transfer your body weight to your hands while lifting your toes. You should then exhale, remaining in the same position for a period of three to four breaths.

Yoga Exercise: What is the Forward Bend?

The forward bend is a seated pose that is considered a basic *asana*. It helps provide a practitioner with a relaxing and easy pose to follow. One of the vital keys in executing the said seated pose is to allow the body to naturally embrace the position instead of forcing it to do so. If the person does the bend properly, it will certain work wonders for the back region. It helps massage the inner organs of the body too, resulting in improved blood circulation.

To start off with this pose, you will have to take deep breaths. When you are getting comfortable, raise your arms upwards in a position that is right next to your head. You should remember to keep the back straight. Lean forward slowly while attempting to catch your feet. The most ideal result of this pose is when you can easily hold your toes within your hands for a certain period. It will be perfect if you can successfully hold your pose for a period of half a minute. When doing this, remember not to let your back arch or to let your legs fold. This means that you will have to put your flexibility into good use. You might even find it difficult to reach the toes with this pose. If this is the case, just try to grab your ankles instead. This should make this pose a lot easier to accomplish. If you want to come out of the said pose, inhale and stretch the body upward slowly until you come back to your initial position.

Your flexibility will really be extremely tested with this pose. In fact, it might even take several weeks before a practitioner can reach the toes and hold this pose for a period of time, even with constant practice. However, you should not get discouraged if your pose is still messy even after several attempts. With this pose, you will have to gradually work at achieving the optimum effects for the body.

Yoga Exercise: What is the Hands-to-Feet Pose?

The hands-to-feet pose is actually a yoga pose that is quite similar to the forward bend, especially in terms of the benefits you can achieve. With the hands-to-feet pose, you will extend and stretch your leg hamstrings to the fullest. You can also increase the flexibility of both your back and spinal column. Another benefit of the hands-to-feet pose is that it increases blood circulation, especially to your head and the rest of the upper body. It is desirable to bend down as far as you can, especially if you can keep your legs straight while doing the hands-to-feet pose. It is necessary to keep the position of your spine straight all throughout this exercise.

To start with the hands-to-feet pose, you should put your hands in the air, with the palms facing one another. Your arms should also be close to the ears, especially when doing a vertical stretch. Keep your feet next to one another. Keep your spine straight by pushing the head in an upward direction. Also, stretch out your entire body in a vertical direction during this process.

From the median region, you should bend forward towards the feet while exhaling. Do not bend your knees too much when doing this, though. Be sure to go as low as possible, but keep your spine straight too. You should then grab your toes, your ankles if not flexible enough, and pull the head toward the legs. Advanced practitioners manage to touch their own shin with their head while in this pose. As one exhales, this should signal you to go one inch lower and closer to your shin.

Coming out of this pose, you should inhale slowly and gently. The movements you executed when entering the said pose should be reversed slowly too. When you are done with stretching the hands above the head, you will have to lower them at your side. After that, relax.

Yoga Exercise: What is the Half Spinal Twist?

Most of the yoga positions these days exist to increase the flexibility of the spinal column. They have things in common such as using a forward-backward position. There may be a few giving you better lateral flexibility, though. A perfect example of one is the half spinal twist. It is the completion of the series of exercises and poses which help develop not only mobility but overall fitness as well. With the said pose, you can easily improve the responses of the spinal nerves. It also helps with the massaging of the internal organs.

It is only natural to keep your spine straight when carrying out the said pose. Then, you should make a circular, sideways motion. Check that the shoulders are kept at a level, especially when a twist is executed. It is vital to have balanced breathing when executing the said pose too. Remember to increase the twist level for every exhalation.

To begin with the half spinal twist, you will have to sit on your knees first. Keep your legs together while resting your buttocks on the sole of the feet. You will have to move the upper body to the right side of your feet, lifting one of your legs in the process to place it over the other one. Your foot will have to go right next to your other leg's knee. With this sequence of actions, you will be twisting your body slowly. Of course, remember to follow your torso's position with both of your hands. Keep your spine straight when doing the said motion for better efficiency.

The next thing to do is to bring the right arm to the left. Remember that this orientation is correct only when the twist performed was oriented to the left side. Your left foot should be held by your hand as your left hand is resting behind you. When twisting, you should not forget to involve your head, all the while looking over your left shoulder.

Yoga Exercise: What is the Head Stand?

The head stand pose is actually considered one of the most beneficial postures for yoga. It will benefit your body and mind a lot. It will be useful in resetting the heart, as well as improving blood circulation and releasing you from back pains.

To be able to execute the head stand pose, you first have to kneel down. It is recommended to have your weight resting on your forearms. You should then wrap your hands around the elbows. Be sure to maintain this position for several seconds. After that, release your hands. Position them in front of the body while keeping your fingers interlocked.

You should then place the top of the head on the ground, all the while keeping the back of your head in your hands. This makes it possible to give the inverted body a firm foundation made up of your hands and elbows. This position will form a tripod. Once you got into this tripod position, you should then straighten your knees while slowly raising your hips.

Bring your feet in, without bending your knees, as close to the head as possible. You should keep your head in a straight line with your spine while pulling in your hips in a manner that prevents the neck from bending.

Bend your knees to your chest, lift the feet off the ground gradually, and move your hips backwards slowly. Take a short break every once in a while. Do not immediately raise your knees. Try to use the abdominal muscles when you are ready to lift the bent knees to the ceiling. Slowly straighten the legs too. Normally, your weight will be on your forearms. To get out of this pose, just reverse the steps you went through.

Yoga Exercise: What is the Yoga Seated Pose?

The sequence of poses is very important for yoga. After all, the preceding poses prepare your body for the next level of intensity involved in the next pose. To those trying out some seated poses, it is best to start it off with *Sukhasana*. This is an easy pose which allows your body to fully adapt to the higher demands of the next positions. You will find *Sukhasana* effective for your neck muscles and upper spinal muscles. You can do *Pranayama* and other similar exercises meant to improve total body flexibility and coordination. Warm up before executing the said poses and be gentle when doing every movement to get good results.

It should already be a given for the person to go for *Sukhasana* when meditating. With this you can maintain a straight spinal position, which can be carried over even when you are done with your yoga exercise. This will offer serenity and introspection as well. Your leg position should alternately be in this posture to avoid getting cramps. While down on the floor with the knees bent, hold your knees within your arms and gently pull them to your chest. The muscles will be stretched with this. After that, release your legs, cross them, and keep the knees close to the ground.

Virasana is the next pose. It is usually referred to as the hero pose. This is similar to the cat pose as well, since you will be sitting on your knees while holding the thighs in a parallel position to one another. Release the pressure from your hands slowly until the hips are lowered to the ground. Mastering this pose may take months and you might also need to have a folded blanket or pillow just to be comfortable when doing this. However, successfully doing *Virasana* will allow better body flexibility if you are able to place the buttocks on the ground with support. Since this is a sitting pose, you should keep your spine straight so draw your abdomen inwards. With *Virasana*, you may need to rest your thighs or knees on your hands. The optimal position in *Virasana* is reached when you can already sit still, with eyes closed, and fall into meditation.

There is the *Paschimothanasana* as well. This is a pose which takes some time to master. It might look easy to execute but it really requires an advanced level of back flexibility, since one is going to stretch all the body muscles starting from the head to the legs. It is a good pose since it helps massage your internal organs. It facilitates blood flow as well. It can easily stimulate the nervous system, which makes it easier to develop better reflexes to any external stimuli. You should have a healthy body to do this pose. If this pose is used in combination with the other yoga poses and balanced diet, you can easily eliminate your fat cells and increase your metabolism rate at the same time. Taking a deep breath when holding this pose and exhale when coming out of this pose. Both your spine and knees should be straight to obtain a maximum stretch.

Yoga Exercise: What are the Shoulder Lifts?

Most practitioners say that they practice yoga for the sake of its health benefits. Indeed, it is a necessity especially when you want to reduce stress and strengthen your muscles. It is a good relaxation and meditation method for you to use nowadays.

Dealing with stress is important, especially since you have lots of daily worries to think of. When it is difficult to concentrate, your thoughts will become more restless and thus they cannot relax anymore.

Stress will affect the areas around the neck and shoulders the most. These are the parts of the body which hold lots of tension. If these are affected, it will cause headaches. Since this is the case, you should do shoulder lifts.

To perform shoulder lifts, you just need to raise one of your shoulders at a time. You can also raise them both simultaneously. Repeat the movements at least five times. You should do this slowly, while keeping the spine straight. Your breathing should be correct too, since this maximizes the exercise's benefits.

When practicing shoulder lifts, you can easily feel relaxed. Tension will slowly leave your body as well. One good thing about this exercise is you can practice this exercise anywhere. The results are always amazing, regardless of where you practice.

Yoga Exercise: What is the Eye Exercise?

Yoga does not only focus on stretches and movements. Most practitioners will also emphasize the importance of eye exercises. Working out the eye muscles prevents possible problems due to tone and muscle vitality loss, which gradually appear as you reach maturity. Eye tension can be reduced if you cultivate the ability to focus at varying distances. They may cause some discomfort.

People recommend the eye exercise since it not only prevents eye illnesses but it improves eyesight as well. It can cure minor eye illnesses so there are many adepts who are interested in this. To proceed with this exercise, use a comfortable seating position. Keep your eyes wide open. Keep your back straight as well as your body relaxed. Your hands should be on top of your knees. During the execution of the said exercise, your body has to remain in the same position. The only body part that should move is your eyes.

Choose two reference points. The first one should be on the wall while the other one is on the floor. Repeatedly shift your sight from one point to the other. This move is just a warm up, however. When feeling prepared, move the eyes as high up as possible and then as far down as you can. Repeat the said moves at least five times, and then blink as quickly as possible to relax the eyes.

Repeat the exercise. This time, you will have to select and use reference points to your right and left, at eye level. Repeat the exercise at least five times. Remember to rest the eye muscles after that.

We Want Your Feedback on This Book!

Our main purpose is to make sure that our readers get value from the books we publish and that they have a good experience with all of our products. We are always working to improve our books and other products with every revision and update.

Every piece of feedback makes a difference in this process. And we would appreciate yours as well - whether it is good or bad.

Please take one minute to let us know what you thought by following this link:
http://checkmatemg.com/feedbackyoga/

www.ingramcontent.com/pod-product-compliance
Lightning Source LLC
Chambersburg PA
CBHW070823290526
45795CB00002B/828

9 781492 891086